Belly Fat Busters for Seniors Cookbook

Over 40 healthy and Flavorful Recipes to Transform Your Health and Shape, a Comprehensive Guide to Losing Weight, Boosting Energy, and Enhancing Wellness

FlavorfulVoyage Books

Copyright © 2024 by FlavorfulVoyage Books

All Right Reserved

No part of this publication may be reproduced, distributed, or transmitted in any form or by any means, including photocopying, recording, or other electronic or mechanical methods, without the prior written permission of the publisher, except in the case of brief quotations embodied in critical reviews and certain other noncommercial uses permitted by copyright law.

Table of Content

Chapter 7: Meal Planning and Prep Weekly Meal Planning Guide

Chapter 8: Success Stories and Testimonials

Chapter 9: Conclusion

Introduction

Hello and welcome to "Belly Fat Busters for Seniors Cookbook: Over 40 Healthy and Flavorful Recipes to Transform Your Health and Shape, a Comprehensive Guide to Losing Weight, Boosting Energy, and Enhancing Wellness." This cookbook is more than just a collection of recipes; it's a complete guide for seniors who want to improve their health, lose belly fat, and live a healthier, more vibrant life in their golden years.

As we age naturally, it becomes more and more clear how important it is to feed our bodies healthy, tasty food. You can do that with the help of this recipe. It focuses on meeting the specific needs of seniors and includes more than 50 carefully chosen recipes that will not only make your taste buds happy but also help you lose weight, get more energy, and improve your general health.

Important Parts of the Cookbook:

1. Transformational Recipes: Tumble into a delicious collection of recipes made to fight belly fat and improve health. From hearty breakfast options to filling dinners and delightful snacks, each recipe is a tasty step toward your health and fitness goals.
2. Comprehensive Nutritional Guide: Learn about the basics of nutrition for adults, with a focus on how important it is to eat a healthy diet full of vital nutrients and limit your portions. This guide serves as a foundation for making educated and health-conscious food decisions.

3. Belly Fat-Busting Ingredients: Uncover the power of adding fiber-rich foods, lean meats, healthy fats, and smart carbs into your daily meals. These carefully picked foods are the cornerstone of the cookbook's approach to healthy living.
4. Practical Tips for Healthy Living: Beyond recipes, learn important insights into keeping a busy and well-rounded lifestyle. Explore the value of regular exercise, effective stress management skills, and the role of hydration in weight control.
5. Meal Planning and Preparation: Simplify the process of planning and making nutritious meals with useful guides, including a weekly meal planning guide, time-saving cooking tips, and advice for efficient food shopping targeted to seniors.
6. Inspiring Success Stories: Draw inspiration from the real-life experiences of seniors who have accepted the principles outlined in this recipe. These success stories are a testament to the changing power of choosing a healthier lifestyle.
7. Encouragement and Closing Thoughts: In the conclusion, find a recap of key concepts, inspiring words to encourage continued commitment to a better lifestyle, and closing thoughts that show thanks for choosing this recipe as a guide on your wellness path.

Embark on this transformative culinary adventure with the "Belly Fat Busters for Seniors Cookbook.". Savor these recipes, your recipe for vibrant health and joyful well-being in your golden years.

Essential Dietary Tips for Seniors

As individuals age, the importance of keeping a healthy and balanced diet becomes increasingly important for general well-being. Healthy food is not just a lifestyle choice; it is a basic component in supporting longevity, controlling chronic conditions, and improving the quality of life, especially for seniors.

1. Nutrient Requirements: Seniors often have changing nutritional needs due to factors such as slower metabolism, changes in digestion, and possible health problems. Therefore, knowing the important nutrients needed for optimal health is vital. Food rich in vitamins, minerals, fiber, and healthy fats supports immune function, bone health, brain function, and energy levels.
2. Chronic Disease Management: Many seniors deal with chronic diseases such as diabetes, heart disease, and osteoporosis. A well-balanced diet plays a key role in controlling these conditions. For instance, a diet low in sodium and saturated fats can add to heart health, while appropriate calcium and vitamin D intake supports bone strength.
3. Weight control: Healthy eating is a cornerstone of successful weight control. Seniors may face challenges related to metabolism and muscle mass

loss, making weight control an important aspect of keeping general health. A varied diet, paired with amount control, helps seniors reach and keep a healthy weight, lowering the risk of obesity-related problems.

4. Energy and Vitality: The right nutrients feed the body and provide the energy needed for daily actions. Seniors who value healthy eating often experience increased vitality and better happiness. Adequate amount of carbohydrates, proteins, and fats ensures prolonged energy levels, adding to a busy and happy lifestyle.

5. Digestive Health: Aging can bring about changes in digestive function, such as lower stomach acid output and slowing digestion. A diet rich in fiber from fruits, veggies, and whole grains improves digestive health, alleviates constipation, and supports a healthy gut microbiome.

6. Brain Function: Research shows a strong link between diet and brain function. Antioxidant-rich foods, omega-3 fatty acids, and a diet low in processed sugars have been linked with a lower chance of cognitive decline in seniors. Understanding these links shows the value of food choices for keeping the brain healthy.

7. Social and Emotional Well-being: Healthy food is not just about physical health; it also adds to social and emotional well-being. Sharing meals with friends and family can create a sense of community and connection, lowering feelings of

loneliness and isolation that some seniors may experience.

Importance of a Balanced Diet

As people gracefully enter their senior years, the importance of keeping a healthy and balanced diet becomes important. Healthy eating is not merely a matter of personal taste; it plays a key role in supporting general well-being, keeping brain function, and avoiding or controlling chronic health conditions that often follow age.

1. Nutrient-Rich Choices: Aging bodies have changing nutritional needs, and making informed choices about what we eat becomes increasingly important. Opting for a diet rich in important nutrients such as vitamins, minerals, fiber, and antioxidants can support immune function, bone health, and energy.
2. Energy and Vitality: Healthy food directly influences energy levels, a key aspect of keeping a busy and happy lifestyle during the golden years. A well-balanced diet provides the necessary fuel for daily tasks, promoting freedom and an improved quality of life.
3. Weight Management: Maintaining a healthy weight is vital to general health, especially for adults. A healthy diet, combined with proper portion control, adds to weight management, lowering the chance of obesity-related health

issues such as diabetes, cardiovascular diseases, and joint problems.

4. Cognitive Health: The effect of diet on cognitive performance is a key factor for seniors. Nutrient-dense foods, especially those rich in omega-3 fatty acids, antioxidants, and vitamins, are linked with better cognitive performance and a reduced chance of cognitive decline.

5. Heart Health: Seniors are often more susceptible to cardiovascular problems, making heart health a concern. Adopting a diet low in saturated and trans fats, sodium, and cholesterol can help greatly to maintain heart health and lower the chance of cardiovascular illnesses.

6. Bone Health: Osteoporosis and bone fractures are typical worries as people age. Calcium and vitamin D-rich foods are important components of a senior's diet, supporting bone health and reducing the risk of fractures.

7. gut Health: Aging can bring about changes in gut function, making fiber-rich foods important for digestive health. Adequate fiber intake helps in digestion, prevents bloating, and supports healthy gut bacteria.

8. Social and Emotional Well-Being: Healthy food is not only about physical health; it also has a deep effect on mental and emotional well-being. Sharing healthy meals with friends and family builds social bonds, while the act of feeding the body adds to a happy mindset.

Chapter 1: Nutritional Basics for Seniors

Essential Nutrients for Seniors

As people age, their nutritional needs face minor yet important changes. Essential nutrients become essential in keeping general health, energy, and resilience against age-related challenges. Here, we dig into the crucial topic of important nutrients for seniors, learning the specific requirements that add to optimal well-being during the golden years.

1. Protein: Protein is a cornerstone food for adults as it supports muscle health, bone density, and immune function. Adequate protein intake becomes increasingly vital for seniors to fight age-related muscle loss (sarcopenia) and support general strength. Good sources of protein for adults include lean meats, chicken, fish, dairy products, beans, and legumes.

2. Calcium and Vitamin D: Calcium is important for keeping bones healthy, and Vitamin D plays a key role in calcium absorption. Together, they help to avoid osteoporosis and fractures, common worries for seniors. Dairy products, leafy veggies, fortified foods, and sunlight exposure are great sources of these nutrients.

3. Fiber: Dietary fiber plays a crucial role in promoting digestive health and avoiding

constipation, a common problem among seniors. Additionally, fiber aids in keeping a healthy weight and controlling blood sugar levels. Whole grains, fruits, veggies, and beans are great sources of dietary fiber.

4. Vitamin B12: Vitamin B12 is important for nerve activity and the production of red blood cells. Aging can affect the body's ability to receive B12 from food, making supplementation or eating of B12-rich foods like meat, fish, eggs, and dairy vital for seniors.

5. Omega-3 Fatty Acids: Omega-3 fatty acids support heart health and brain function, giving protection against conditions like heart disease and cognitive decline. Fatty fish (salmon, trout), flaxseeds, chia seeds, and walnuts are great sources of omega-3s.

6. Potassium: Seniors need sufficient potassium for maintaining proper heart function, controlling blood pressure, and supporting general cardiovascular health. Bananas, oranges, potatoes, spinach, and beans are good food sources of potassium.

7. Antioxidants (Vitamins C and E): Antioxidants play a part in neutralizing free radicals, possibly reducing the chance of chronic diseases linked with aging. Fruits, veggies, nuts, and seeds rich in vitamins C and E add to antioxidant intake.

8. Magnesium: Magnesium is important for keeping muscle and nerve function, supporting the immune system, and improving bone health. Whole grains,

nuts, seeds, and green leafy veggies are great sources of magnesium.

9. Water: Staying properly hydrated becomes increasingly important for seniors to support digestion, kidney function, and general hydration. Drinking water and eating hydrating foods like fruits and veggies are important.

Ensuring a well-rounded and nutrient-dense diet is vital for adults to thrive in their later years.

Portion Control and Meal Planning

Maintaining a healthy lifestyle, especially for seniors, involves more than just picking nutrient-rich foods—it takes a mindful approach to portion control and smart meal planning. These two components play a crucial role in controlling weight, supporting general health, and ensuring a well-balanced diet.

1. Portion Control: Portion control is the practice of moderating the amount of food eaten at one time. For adults, who may have different nutritional needs and metabolism rates, understanding serving sizes is important. Here are key factors to consider:
   - Tailoring Portions to Individual Needs: Seniors often require fewer calories than younger people. Adjusting meal sizes to match individual exercise levels, metabolism, and health goals is important for keeping a healthy weight.

- Listening to Hunger and Fullness Cues: Learning to notice and react to feelings of hunger and fullness helps seniors avoid overeating. Mindful eating allows for a more enjoyable and satisfying meal experience.
- Balancing Macronutrients: Achieving a healthy distribution of macronutrients (proteins, fats, and carbs) within each meal supports satiety and provides prolonged energy throughout the day.

2. Meal Planning: Meal planning goes hand in hand with portion control, giving an organized approach to organizing and making well-rounded, nutritious meals. Here's why meal planning is particularly helpful for seniors:

- Ensuring Nutrient Adequacy: Seniors often face challenges such as reduced hunger or trouble making meals. Meal planning allows for the creation of well-balanced and nutrient-dense dishes, ensuring that important vitamins and minerals are added to daily meals.
- Promoting Consistency: Consistency in meal time and substance helps control blood sugar levels and supports digestive health. Seniors can benefit from a schedule that includes planned meals and snacks throughout the day.
- Reducing Food Waste: Planning meals in advance helps seniors to buy items in suitable quantities, minimizing food waste.

This not only adds to cost savings but also fits with sustainable and eco-friendly practices.

- Adapting to Dietary Restrictions: Many seniors may have dietary restrictions or specific health issues that require careful thought. Meal planning allows the modification of meals to meet individual needs, ensuring optimal nutrition while sticking to any recommended nutritional standards.

Practical Tips for Seniors:

- Smaller, Frequent Meals: Instead of three large meals, try incorporating smaller, more frequent meals throughout the day to control hunger and keep energy levels.
- Colorful Plate Strategy: Aim for a colorful plate by including a range of fruits and veggies. This not only improves visual appeal but also provides a varied range of nutrients.
- Mindful Eating Practices: Slow down, enjoy each bite, and pay attention to hunger and fullness cues. This mindful method creates a more aware and enjoyable eating experience.
- Utilize Technology: Seniors can explore meal planning apps or tools that ease the process, helping them organize recipes,

make shopping lists, and track nutritional content.

Chapter 2: Belly Fat-Busting Ingredients

Incorporating Fiber-Rich Foods

Incorporating fiber-rich foods into your diet is a key component of keeping general health and well-being. Dietary fiber, found in plant-based foods, plays a crucial role in supporting digestive health, controlling weight, and lowering the risk of different chronic diseases.

Benefits of Fiber:

1. Digestive Health: Fiber adds bulk to the diet, promoting normal bowel movements and avoiding constipation. It also helps keep a good balance of gut bacteria.
2. Weight Management: High-fiber foods are often lower in calories and more filling, making them a useful component of weight management and hunger control.
3. Blood Sugar Control: Fiber helps manage blood sugar levels by slowing the uptake of sugar. This is particularly beneficial for people with diabetes or those at risk of getting the condition.
4. Heart Health: Soluble fiber, found in oats, beans, and veggies, can help lower cholesterol levels, lowering the risk of heart disease.
5. Satiety and Weight Loss: Fiber-rich foods add to a feeling of fullness, reducing the chance of overeating and aiding in weight loss efforts.

Sources of Dietary Fiber:

1. Whole Grains: Include whole grains like oats, brown rice, quinoa, and whole wheat in your diet for a large fiber boost.
2. Fruits and veggies: Aim for a colorful range of fruits and veggies, as they are naturally rich in fiber, vitamins, and minerals.
3. Legumes: Beans, lentils, and beans are great sources of both soluble and insoluble fiber.
4. Nuts and Seeds: Almonds, chia seeds, flaxseeds, and other nuts and seeds are healthy snacks that add to your daily fiber intake.
5. veggies with Skin: Leave the skin on veggies like potatoes and carrots, as it includes useful fiber.

Choosing Lean Proteins

Choosing lean meats is a crucial part of a healthy and balanced diet. Lean proteins are nutrient-dense sources of important amino acids, vital for keeping muscle mass, supporting immune function, and promoting general well-being. Unlike fatty cuts of meat, lean proteins contain smaller amounts of saturated fats, making them heart-friendly and suitable for those looking to control their weight.

Examples of lean proteins include skinless chicken, lean cuts of beef or pork, fish, tofu, beans, and low-fat dairy products. Incorporating these sources into your diet provides the body with high-quality protein without extra calories or bad fats. Moreover, lean proteins add to a feeling of fullness, aiding in weight control and preventing overeating.

When picking lean proteins, it's important to consider cooking methods. Grilling, baking, broiling, and steaming are better alternatives to frying, as they help keep the protein's nutritional value while minimizing added fats. Making conscious choices about the protein sources in your meals is an easy yet impactful way to improve your diet, supporting your general health and wellness.

Healthy Fats for Seniors

In the world of senior nutrition, knowing the significance of incorporating healthy fats into one's diet is crucial. Healthy fats play a crucial role in supporting general well-being, especially as people age. These fats are important for keeping cognitive function, supporting heart health, and helping in the absorption of fat-soluble vitamins.

Key Points:

1. Brain Health: Omega-3 fatty acids, found in fatty fish like salmon and trout, as well as in nuts and seeds, are known for their brain-boosting qualities. Including these healthy fats in a senior's diet may add to cognitive health and possibly lower the risk of age-related cognitive decline.

2. Heart Health: Monounsaturated and polyunsaturated fats, found in olive oil, bananas, and nuts, have been associated with heart health. These fats can help control cholesterol levels, lower inflammation, and support cardiovascular well-being.
3. Joint Health: Omega-3 fatty acids also show anti-inflammatory qualities, which can be helpful for seniors dealing with joint pain or arthritis. Foods like flaxseeds, chia seeds, and walnuts are great sources.
4. Vitamin uptake: Healthy fats help in the uptake of fat-soluble vitamins A, D, E, and K. Including a modest amount of healthy fats in meals helps seniors improve the nutritional benefits of their diet.
5. Weight Management: Contrary to the misconception that all fats lead to weight gain, healthy fats can add to satiety and help seniors keep a healthy weight. This is especially important as keeping an acceptable weight is linked to various aspects of overall health.

Smart Carbohydrate Choices

In the world of nutrition, making smart carbohydrate choices is a key aspect of supporting general health and well-being. Unlike simple carbohydrates, which are quickly digested and can cause spikes in blood sugar levels, smart carbohydrates are complicated and provide longer energy while giving important nutrients.

These smart carbohydrate choices include whole grains, beans, fruits, and veggies. Whole grains, such as quinoa, brown rice, and oats, are rich in fiber, improving gut health and adding to a feeling of fullness. Legumes, such as beans and lentils, not only provide a good source of complex carbohydrates but are also packed with protein and important minerals.

Fruits and veggies, with their natural sugars and fiber levels, are excellent smart carbohydrate picks. They offer a range of vitamins, minerals, and enzymes, supporting general health and giving a steady release of energy throughout the day.

By choosing smart carbohydrate choices, people can keep stable energy levels, support weight control, and add to long-term health goals. This approach to food is an important part of a healthy and nutritious diet

Chapter 3: Flavorful and Healthy Breakfast Recipes

Berry Bliss Fiber-Packed Smoothie Bowl:

Ingredients:

- 1 cup mixed berries (strawberries, blueberries, raspberries)
- 1 ripe banana, frozen
- 1/2 cup Greek yogurt
- 1/4 cup rolled oats
- 1 tablespoon chia seeds
- 1 tablespoon honey or maple syrup (optional)
- 1/2 cup almond milk
- Toppings: Sliced strawberries, blueberries, granola, and a sprinkle of chia seeds.

Instructions:

- In a mixer, add the mixed berries, frozen banana, Greek yogurt, rolled oats, chia seeds, honey (if using), and almond milk.
- Blend until smooth and creamy, adding more almond milk if needed to hit your desired consistency.
- Pour the juice into a bowl.
- Top with sliced strawberries, blueberries, granola, and a sprinkle of chia seeds.
- Enjoy with a spoon and enjoy the burst of tastes and textures!

Tropical Paradise Fiber-Packed Smoothie Bowl:

Ingredients:

- 1 cup frozen mango chunks
- 1/2 cup pineapple chunks
- 1/2 banana
- 1/2 cup spinach leaves (for extra fiber and nutrients)
- 1/4 cup plain yogurt
- 1 tablespoon flaxseeds
- 1 tablespoon coconut flakes
- 1/2 cup coconut water or almond milk
- Toppings: Sliced kiwi, passion fruit seeds, granola, and a sprinkle of coconut flakes.

Instructions:

- In a blender, mix the frozen mango chunks, pineapple chunks, banana, spinach, normal yogurt, flaxseeds, and coconut water or almond milk.
- Blend until smooth and creamy.
- Pour the juice into a bowl.
- Top with sliced kiwi, passion fruit seeds, granola, and a sprinkle of coconut flakes.
- Dive into this tropical treat and enjoy the nutrient-rich goodness!

Green Goddess Fiber-Packed Smoothie Bowl:

Ingredients:

- 1 cup kale leaves, tips removed
- 1/2 cup cucumber, peeled and chopped
- 1/2 avocado
- 1/2 green apple, cored
- 1 tablespoon hemp seeds
- 1 tablespoon spirulina powder (optional)
- 1/2 cup coconut water or water
- Toppings: Sliced green apple, kiwi bits, pumpkin seeds, and a drizzle of honey.

Instructions:

- In a mixer, add the kale leaves, cucumber, avocado, green apple, hemp seeds, spirulina powder (if using), and coconut water or water.
- Blend until smooth and bright green.
- Pour the juice into a bowl.
- Top with chopped green apple, kiwi bits, pumpkin seeds, and a drizzle of honey.
- Delight in the freshness and nutrient-packed goodness of this Green Goddess smoothie bowl!

Chocolate Peanut Butter Banana Bowl:

Ingredients:

- 2 ripe bananas
- 2 tablespoons cocoa powder
- 2 tablespoons peanut butter
- 1/2 cup Greek yogurt
- 1 tablespoon flaxseeds
- 1/2 cup milk (dairy or plant-based)

Toppings:

- Sliced banana
- Crushed peanuts
- Dark chocolate flakes
- Drizzle of peanut butter

Instructions

- Peel and slice the ripe bananas.
- In a blender, combine the sliced bananas, cocoa powder, peanut butter, Greek yogurt, flaxseeds, and milk.
- Blend the ingredients until you achieve a smooth and creamy consistency. Add more milk if needed to reach your desired thickness.
- Pour the chocolate peanut butter banana mixture into a bowl.
- Decorate the bowl with sliced banana pieces, crushed peanuts, and dark chocolate shavings.
- Finish off your delicious bowl with a generous drizzle of peanut butter.

Mixed Berry Protein Bowl:

Ingredients:

- cup mixed berries (strawberries, blueberries, blackberries)
- 1/2 cup cottage cheese
- 1 scoop vanilla protein powder
- 1 tablespoon almond butter
- 1/2 cup unsweetened almond milk
- 1 tablespoon chia seeds

Toppings:

- Granola
- Sliced strawberries
- Chopped nuts (walnuts or almonds)
- Drizzle of honey

Instructions

- Place all the drink ingredients in a blender.
- Blend until smooth and creamy.
- Pour the juice into a bowl.
- Arrange items as asked.
- Enjoy with a spoon and enjoy the fiber-packed goodness!

Whole Grain Pancakes with Fresh Fruit

Classic Whole Grain Pancakes with Mixed Berries:

Ingredients:

- 1 cup whole wheat flour
- 1 tablespoon sugar
- 1 teaspoon baking powder
- 1/2 teaspoon baking soda
- 1 cup buttermilk
- 1 large egg
- 2 tablespoons melted butter
- Mixed berries (strawberries, blueberries, raspberries) for topping

Instructions:

- In a bowl, mix flour, sugar, baking powder, and baking soda.
- In another bowl, mix buttermilk, egg, and melted butter.
- Combine wet and dry ingredients until just mixed.
- Heat a pan or pot over medium heat and pour batter onto it.
- Cook until bubbles form, flip, and cook until golden brown.
- Serve topped with a large handful of mixed berries.

Banana Walnut Whole Grain Pancakes:

Ingredients:

- 1 cup whole-grain pancake mix
- 1 ripe banana, mashed
- 1/2 cup chopped walnuts
- 1 cup milk
- 1 large egg
- 2 tablespoons maple syrup
- Sliced bananas for garnish

Instructions:

- Combine pancake mix, mashed banana, chopped walnuts, milk, egg, and maple syrup.
- Mix until just mixed.
- Cook on a grill or pan until golden brown on both sides.
- Garnish with sliced bananas and an extra drizzle of maple syrup.

Blueberry Almond Whole Grain Pancakes:

Ingredients:

- 1 cup whole wheat flour
- 1 tablespoon sugar
- 1 teaspoon baking powder
- 1/2 teaspoon baking soda
- 1 cup almond milk
- 1 large egg
- 1/2 cup fresh blueberries

- Sliced almonds for topping

Instructions:

- Whisk together flour, sugar, baking powder, and baking soda.
- In a different bowl, mix almond milk and egg.
- Combine wet and dry ingredients, and fold in blueberries.
- Cook pancakes until golden brown, and top with sliced nuts.

Apple Cinnamon Whole Grain Pancakes:

Ingredients:

- 1 cup whole-grain pancake mix
- 1/2 cup grated apple
- 1/2 teaspoon ground cinnamon
- 1 cup milk
- 1 large egg
- Sliced apples for garnish

Instructions:

- Mix pancake mix, chopped apple, cinnamon, milk, and egg.
- Cook on a pan until golden brown.
- Garnish with cut apples and a sprinkle of cinnamon.

Orange Cranberry Whole Grain Pancakes:

Ingredients:

- 1 cup whole wheat flour
- 1 tablespoon sugar
- 1 teaspoon baking powder
- 1/2 teaspoon baking soda
- 1 cup orange juice
- Zest of one orange
- 1 large egg
- 1/2 cup fresh cranberries

Instructions:

- Combine the dry ingredients: flour, sugar, baking powder, and baking soda. 2. In another bowl, mix orange juice, orange zest, and egg.
- Combine wet and dry ingredients, and fold in cranberries.
- Cook until pancakes are golden brown and serve with a drizzle of honey.

Greek Yogurt Parfait with Nuts and Berries

Classic Greek Yogurt Parfait:

- Ingredients:
- 1 cup Greek yogurt
- 1/2 cup granola

- 1/2 cup mixed berries (strawberries, blueberries, raspberries)
- 2 tablespoons honey
- 2 tablespoons chopped nuts (almonds, walnuts)

Instructions:

- In a glass or bowl, layer Greek yogurt at the bottom.
- Add a layer of cereal on top of the yogurt.
- Sprinkle a handful of mixed berries over the granola.
- Drizzle honey over the berries.
- Repeat the steps until the jar is filled.
- Finish with a nutty crunch: top with chopped nuts.
- Serve quickly and enjoy a lovely Greek yogurt dessert.

Tropical Twist Greek Yogurt Parfait:

Ingredients:

- 1 cup Greek yogurt
- 1/2 cup pineapple chunks
- 1/2 cup mango cubes
- 2 tablespoons shredded coconut
- 2 tablespoons granola
- Mint leaves for garnish (optional)

Instructions:

- Begin by putting Greek yogurt in a serving glass or bowl.
- Add a layer of pineapple bits and mango cubes.
- Sprinkle chopped coconut over the fruit layer.
- Add a layer of oats for extra grit.
- Repeat the steps until the jar is filled.
- Garnish with mint leaves if wanted.
- Serve cold and enjoy the tropical tastes.

Berry Nut Bliss Greek Yogurt Parfait:

Ingredients:

- 1 cup Greek yogurt
- 1/2 cup mixed berries (strawberries, blueberries, blackberries)
- 2 tablespoons chopped nuts (pecans, almonds)
- 1 tablespoon chia seeds
- 1 tablespoon honey

Instructions:

- Start by putting Greek yogurt at the bottom of a glass.
- Add a layer of mixed berries over the yogurt.
- Sprinkle chopped nuts and chia seeds over the berries.
- Drizzle honey over the layers for sweetness.
- Repeat the process until the jar is full.
- Allow the chia seeds to soak for a few minutes.

- Enjoy this nutrient-packed berry and nut Greek yogurt dish.

Chocolate Berry Greek Yogurt Parfait:

Ingredients:

- 1 cup Greek yogurt
- 2 tablespoons chocolate powder
- 1/2 cup mixed berries (strawberries, raspberries)
- 2 tablespoons chocolate chips
- 1/4 cup granola

Instructions:

- In a bowl, mix Greek yogurt with chocolate powder.
- Begin piling with the chocolate Greek yogurt at the bottom.
- Add a layer of mixed berries over the chocolate yogurt.
- Sprinkle chocolate chips for extra pleasure.
- Top with a layer of granola for crunch.
- Repeat the steps until the jar is full.
- Dive into the rich tastes of this chocolate-infused Greek yogurt treat.

Maple Pecan Greek Yogurt Parfait:

Ingredients:

- 1 cup Greek yogurt
- 2 tablespoons maple syrup
- 1/2 cup sliced strawberries
- 1/4 cup chopped pecans
- 2 tablespoons granola

Instructions:

- Drizzle maple syrup into Greek yogurt and mix well.
- Layer the maple-infused yogurt at the bottom of a glass.
- Add a layer of sliced strawberries over the yogurt.
- Sprinkle chopped nuts for a delicious nutty taste.
- Top with a layer of granola for extra crunch.
- Repeat the steps until the jar is full.
- Savor the sweetness of this maple and pecan Greek yogurt dish.

Chapter 4: Lunchtime Delights

Grilled Chicken Salad with Avocado:

Ingredients:

- 2 boneless, skinless chicken breasts
- Salt and pepper to taste
- 2 tablespoons olive oil
- 6 cups mixed salad greens
- 1 cup cherry tomatoes, halved
- 1 cucumber, sliced
- 1 avocado, sliced
- 1/4 cup feta cheese, crumbled
- Balsamic vinegar sauce

Instructions:

- Season the chicken breasts lightly with salt and pepper, ensuring even distribution.
- Heat olive oil in a grill pan over medium-high heat until shimmering and lightly smoking.
- Grill chicken for 6-8 minutes per side or until fully cooked.
- Let the chicken rest for a few minutes, then slice it into strips.
- In a large bowl, toss together the salad leaves, cherry tomatoes, onion, and avocado.
- Top the salad with grilled chicken strips.
- Sprinkle feta cheese over the salad.
- Drizzle balsamic vinegar sauce over the salad and mix gently.

- Serve quickly for a refreshing and filling lunch.

Quinoa and Vegetable Stuffed Peppers:

Ingredients:

- 4 bell peppers, split and seeds removed
- 1 cup quinoa, cooked
- 1 (15 oz) can black beans, drained and rinsed
- 1 cup corn kernels, either fresh or frozen
- 1 cup cherry tomatoes, diced
- 1/2 cup red onion, roughly chopped
- 1 cup shredded cheddar cheese
- 1 teaspoon cumin
- Salt and pepper to taste
- Fresh parsley for garnish

Instructions:

- Preheat the oven to 375°F (190°C).
- In a big bowl, mix cooked rice, black beans, corn, cherry tomatoes, red onion, cumin, salt, and pepper.
- Stuff each bell pepper half with the rice filling.
- Top with shredded cheddar cheese.
- Place stuffed peppers on a baking sheet and bake for 25-30 minutes or until peppers are soft.
- Garnish with fresh cilantro before serving.

Salmon and Asparagus Wraps:

Ingredients:

- 4 salmon chunks
- 1 bunch asparagus, cut
- 2 tablespoons olive oil
- 1 lemon, sliced
- Salt and pepper to taste
- 4 whole-grain sandwiches

Instructions:

- Preheat the oven to 400°F (200°C).
- Lay out the asparagus and salmon pieces on a baking sheet.
- Third, add olive oil and salt and pepper to taste.
- Lay lemon slices over the salmon.
- Bake for 15-20 minutes or until the salmon is cooked through.
- Warm the whole-grain wraps.
- Assemble wraps with baked salmon and asparagus.
- Serve immediately.

Turkey and Vegetable Stir-Fry:

Ingredients:

- 1 pound ground turkey
- 2 cups broccoli florets
- 1 bell pepper, thinly sliced
- 1 carrot, julienned

- 2 tablespoons soy sauce
- 1 tablespoon hoisin sauce
- 1 tablespoon sesame oil
- 2 garlic cloves, minced
- 1 teaspoon ginger, grated
- Cooked brown rice for serving

Instructions:

- In a wok or large skillet, brown the ground turkey over medium-high heat.
- Add broccoli, bell pepper, and carrot to the skillet.
- In a small bowl, mix soy sauce, hoisin sauce, sesame oil, garlic, and ginger.
- Pour the sauce over the turkey and vegetables, stirring to combine.
- Cook for an additional 5-7 minutes until the vegetables are tender.
- Serve the stir-fry over cooked brown rice.

Vegetarian Chili with Beans and Greens:

Ingredients:

- 2 cans of black beans, drained and rinsed
- 1 can diced tomatoes
- 1 cup corn kernels (fresh or frozen)
- 1 onion, diced
- 2 bell peppers, diced
- 2 cups kale, chopped
- 2 tablespoons chili powder

- 1 teaspoon cumin
- Salt and pepper to taste
- Greek yogurt and chopped green onions for topping

Instructions:

- In a large pot, sauté onion and bell peppers until softened.
- Add black beans, diced tomatoes, corn, kale, chili powder, cumin, salt, and pepper.
- Stir well and bring to a simmer.
- Cover and cook for 20-25 minutes until flavors meld.
- Serve the vegetarian chili topped with a dollop of Greek yogurt and chopped green onions.

Caprese Chicken Salad:

Ingredients:

- 2 boneless, skinless chicken breasts
- Salt and pepper to taste
- 1 tablespoon olive oil
- 1 cup cherry tomatoes, halved
- 1 cup fresh mozzarella balls
- Fresh basil leaves
- Balsamic glaze for drizzling

Instructions:

- Put salt and pepper on the chicken breasts.

- Heat olive oil in a skillet over medium-high heat.
- Cook chicken for 6-8 minutes per side or until fully cooked.
- Slice chicken into thin strips.
- In a bowl, combine cherry tomatoes, mozzarella balls, and sliced chicken.
- Add fresh basil leaves and drizzle with balsamic glaze.
- Toss gently and serve.

Sweet Potato and Chickpea Buddha Bowl:

Ingredients:

- 2 sweet potatoes, cubed
- 1 can chickpeas, drained and rinsed
- 1 tablespoon olive oil
- 1 teaspoon cumin
- 1 teaspoon smoked paprika
- Salt and pepper to taste
- Quinoa or brown rice for serving
- Avocado slices for garnish

Instructions:

- Preheat the oven to 400°F (200°C).
- Toss sweet potatoes and chickpeas with olive oil, cumin, smoked paprika, salt, and pepper.
- Roast in the oven for 25-30 minutes until golden and crispy.
- Serve over quinoa or brown rice.

- Garnish with avocado slices.

Pesto Zoodle Bowl with Grilled Shrimp:

Ingredients:

- Zucchini, spiralized into noodles
- 1 pound shrimp, peeled and deveined
- 2 tablespoons pesto sauce
- Cherry tomatoes, halved
- Pine nuts for garnish
- Fresh basil leaves

Instructions:

- Grill shrimp until cooked through.
- In a pan, sauté zucchini noodles until just tender.
- Toss zoodles with pesto sauce.
- Arrange zoodles in bowls and top with grilled shrimp and cherry tomatoes.
- Garnish with pine nuts and fresh basil leaves.

Mediterranean Quinoa Salad:

Ingredients:

- 1 cup quinoa, cooked
- 1 cucumber, diced
- 1 cup cherry tomatoes, halved
- 1/2 red onion, finely chopped
- Kalamata olives, sliced

- Feta cheese, crumbled
- Fresh parsley, chopped
- Lemon vinaigrette dressing

Instructions:

- In a large bowl, combine cooked quinoa, cucumber, cherry tomatoes, red onion, olives, and feta cheese.
- Add the lemon vinaigrette sauce and gently toss the salad.
- Sprinkle fresh parsley on top.
- Serve chilled.

Turkey Avocado Wrap:

Ingredients:

- Sliced turkey breast
- Whole-grain wraps
- Avocado, sliced
- Tomato, sliced
- Lettuce leaves
- Hummus
- Dijon mustard

Instructions:

- Lay out a whole-grain wrap on a flat surface.
- Spread a layer of hummus and Dijon mustard on the wrap.
- Arrange sliced turkey, avocado, tomato, and lettuce leaves in the center.

- Fold in the sides and roll the wrap tightly.
- Slice in half and serve.

Chapter 5: Satisfying Dinners

Grilled Lemon Herb Salmon with Roasted Vegetables:

Ingredients:

- 4 salmon chunks
- 1 lemon (zested and juiced)
- 2 tablespoons olive oil
- 2 cloves garlic (minced)
- 1 teaspoon dried thyme
- 1 teaspoon dried rosemary
- Salt and black pepper to taste
- 1 pound mixed vegetables (e.g., bell peppers, zucchini, cherry tomatoes)

Instructions:

- Warm up the oven or grill over medium-high heat.
- In a bowl, mix the lemon zest, lemon juice, olive oil, minced garlic, thyme, rosemary, salt, and pepper to create a marinade.
- Brush the salmon fillets with the marinade and let them sit for 15-20 minutes.
- Thread the mixed vegetables onto skewers and brush them with the remaining marinade.
- Grill the salmon for 4-5 minutes per side or bake in the oven at 400°F (200°C) for about 15-20 minutes, until the salmon is cooked through.
- Grill or roast the vegetable skewers until they are tender and slightly charred.

- Serve the grilled salmon on a bed of roasted vegetables for a satisfying and nutritious dinner.

Turkey and Vegetable Stir-Fry:

Ingredients:

- 1 pound lean ground turkey
- 2 tablespoons soy sauce
- 1 tablespoon sesame oil
- 1 tablespoon ginger (minced)
- 2 cloves garlic (minced)
- 1 cup broccoli florets
- 1 bell pepper (sliced)
- 1 carrot (julienned)
- 1 cup snap peas
- 2 green onions (sliced)
- Cooked brown rice or quinoa for serving

Instructions:

- In a wok or large skillet, brown the ground turkey over medium-high heat.
- In a small bowl, mix soy sauce and sesame oil. Set aside.
- Add ginger and garlic to the browned turkey, sautéing until fragrant.
- Add broccoli, bell pepper, carrot, and snap peas to the wok. Stir-fry for 5-7 minutes until vegetables are crisp-tender.

- Pour the soy sauce mixture over the turkey and vegetables, stirring well to coat.
- Cook for an additional 2-3 minutes until everything is heated through.
- Serve the stir-fry over cooked brown rice or quinoa, garnished with sliced green onions.

Baked Cod with Lemon and Herbs:

Ingredients:

- 4 cod fillets
- 2 tablespoons olive oil
- 2 tablespoons fresh lemon juice
- 1 teaspoon dried oregano
- 1 teaspoon dried thyme
- 1 teaspoon garlic powder
- Salt and black pepper to taste
- Lemon wedges for serving

Instructions:

- Preheat the oven to 400°F (200°C) and grease a baking dish.
- Place the cod fillets in the baking dish.
- In a small bowl, mix olive oil, lemon juice, oregano, thyme, garlic powder, salt, and pepper.
- Brush the cod fillets with the lemon and herb mixture, ensuring they are well-coated.
- Bake in the preheated oven for 15-20 minutes or until the fish flakes easily with a fork.

- Serve the baked cod with additional lemon wedges for a fresh and satisfying dinner option.

Quinoa and Vegetable Stuffed Peppers:

Ingredients:

- 4 bell peppers (halved and seeds removed)
- 1 cup quinoa (cooked)
- 1 can of black beans, washed and set aside
- 1 cup corn kernels (fresh or frozen)
- 1 cup cherry tomatoes (halved)
- 1 cup shredded cheddar cheese
- 1 teaspoon ground cumin
- 1 teaspoon chili powder
- Salt and black pepper to taste
- Fresh parsley for garnish

Instructions:

- Preheat the oven to 375°F (190°C).
- In a bowl, mix cooked quinoa, black beans, corn, cherry tomatoes, cheese, cumin, chili powder, salt, and pepper.
- Stuff each bell pepper half with the rice filling.
- Place stuffed peppers in a baking dish and bake for 25-30 minutes or until peppers are tender.
- Garnish with fresh cilantro and serve.

Chicken and Vegetable Skewers with Peanut Sauce:

Ingredients:

- 1 pound boneless, skinless chicken breasts (cut into chunks)
- 1 bell pepper (cut into chunks)
- 1 red onion (cut into chunks)
- 1 zucchini (sliced)
- Wooden skewers (pre-soaked)
- 1/2 cup peanut butter
- 2 tablespoons soy sauce
- 1 tablespoon honey
- 1 tablespoon lime juice
- 1 teaspoon ginger (minced)
- 1 garlic clove (minced)
- Crushed red pepper flakes (optional)

Instructions:

- Preheat the grill or grill pan.
- Thread chicken, bell pepper, red onion, and zucchini onto skewers.
- In a small bowl, whisk together peanut butter, soy sauce, honey, lime juice, ginger, garlic, and red pepper flakes (if using) to make the sauce.
- Grill the skewers for 8-10 minutes, turning occasionally, until the chicken is cooked through.
- Serve the skewers drizzled with peanut sauce.

Sweet Potato and Chickpea Curry:

Ingredients:

- 2 big sweet potatoes, cut up
- 1 can chickpeas (drained and rinsed)
- 1 onion (chopped)
- 2 cloves garlic (minced)
- 1 can coconut milk
- 1 can diced tomatoes
- 2 tablespoons curry powder
- 1 teaspoon ground cumin
- 1 teaspoon ground coriander
- Salt and black pepper to taste
- Fresh parsley for garnish

Instructions:

- In a large pot, sauté onion and garlic until softened.
- Add sweet potatoes, chickpeas, coconut milk, diced tomatoes, curry powder, cumin, coriander, salt, and pepper.
- Simmer for 20-25 minutes or until sweet potatoes are tender.
- Garnish with fresh cilantro before serving.

Spinach and Feta Stuffed Chicken Breast:

Ingredients:

- 4 boneless, skinless chicken breasts
- 2 cups fresh spinach (chopped)
- 1/2 cup feta cheese (crumbled)
- 1 teaspoon dried oregano
- 1 teaspoon garlic powder

- Salt and black pepper to taste
- Olive oil for cooking

Instructions:

- Preheat the oven to 400°F (200°C).
- In a bowl, mix chopped spinach, feta, oregano, garlic powder, salt, and pepper.
- Cut a pocket into each chicken breast and stuff with the spinach and feta mixture.
- Secure with toothpicks if needed.
- Heat olive oil in an oven-safe skillet and sear the chicken on both sides until golden.
- When the chicken is done, put the pan in the oven and bake for 20 to 25 minutes.

Mediterranean Chickpea Salad:

Ingredients:

- 2 cans chickpeas (drained and rinsed)
- 1 cucumber (diced)
- 1 cup cherry tomatoes (halved)
- 1 red onion (finely chopped)
- 1 and a half cups of sliced Kalamata olives
- 1/2 cup feta cheese (crumbled)
- 1/4 cup fresh parsley (chopped)
- 3 tablespoons olive oil
- 2 tablespoons red wine vinegar
- 1 teaspoon dried oregano
- Salt and black pepper to taste

Instructions:

- In a large bowl, combine chickpeas, cucumber, cherry tomatoes, red onion, olives, feta, and parsley.
- In a small bowl, whisk together olive oil, red wine vinegar, oregano, salt, and pepper to make the dressing.
- Pour the sauce over the salad and toss to mix.
- Chill in the freezer for at least thirty minutes before serving.

Shrimp and Avocado Salad:

Ingredients:

- 1 pound shrimp (peeled and deveined)
- 2 avocados (diced)
- 1 cup cherry tomatoes (halved)
- 1 cucumber (sliced)
- 1/4 cup red onion (finely chopped)
- 1/4 cup cilantro (chopped)
- 2 tablespoons olive oil
- 2 tablespoons lime juice
- 1 teaspoon cumin
- Salt and black pepper to taste

Instructions:

- Season shrimp with cumin, salt, and pepper.

- Heat olive oil in a skillet and cook shrimp until pink and opaque.
- In a large bowl, combine cooked shrimp, diced avocados, cherry tomatoes, cucumber, red onion, and cilantro.
- In a small bowl, whisk together lime juice, olive oil, salt, and pepper to make the dressing.
- Drizzle the sauce over the bowl of salad and shake gently before serving.

Eggplant and Chickpea Bake:

Ingredients:

- 1 large eggplant (sliced)
- 1 can chickpeas (drained and rinsed)
- 2 cups tomato sauce
- 1 cup mozzarella cheese (shredded)
- 1/4 cup Parmesan cheese (grated)
- 2 tablespoons olive oil
- 1 teaspoon dried basil
- 1 teaspoon dried oregano
- Salt and black pepper to taste

Instructions:

- Preheat the oven to 375°F (190°C).
- In a baking dish, layer sliced eggplant, chickpeas, and tomato sauce.
- Sprinkle with mozzarella and Parmesan cheese.

- Drizzle olive oil over the top and sprinkle with dried basil, dried oregano, salt, and pepper.
- Bake for 30-35 minutes or until the cheese is melted and bubbly.

Chapter 6: Snacks and Treats

Sweet Potato and Rosemary Baked Fries:

Ingredients:

- Sweet potatoes, Sliced and cut into fries
- Olive oil
- Fresh rosemary, finely chopped
- Salt and pepper to taste

Instructions:

- Preheat oven to 400°F (200°C).
- Toss sweet potato fries in olive oil, rosemary, salt, and pepper.
- Spread on a baking sheet in a single layer.
- Bake for 25-30 minutes or until crispy, flipping halfway through.

Caprese Skewers with Balsamic Glaze:

Ingredients:

- Cherry tomatoes
- Fresh mozzarella balls
- Fresh basil leaves
- Balsamic glaze
- Skewers

Instructions:

- Thread a tomato, mozzarella ball, and basil leaf onto each skewer.
- Arrange on a serving platter.
- Drizzle with balsamic glaze just before serving.

Oatmeal Energy Bites:

Ingredients:

- Rolled oats
- Peanut butter
- Honey
- Chia seeds
- Mini chocolate chips

Instructions:

- In a bowl, mix rolled oats, peanut butter, honey, chia seeds, and mini chocolate chips.
- Form small balls using the mixture.
- Place in the refrigerator for at least 30 minutes before serving. Enjoy as a quick energy-boosting snack!

Avocado and Black Bean Salsa:

Ingredients:

- Ripe avocados, diced
- Black beans, drained and washed
- Red onion, roughly chopped

- Cilantro, chopped
- Lime juice

Instructions:

- Combine avocados, black beans, red onion, and cilantro in a bowl.
- Drizzle with lime juice and mix gently. Serve with taco chips.

Cucumber Hummus Bites:

- Ingredients:
- Cucumber, cut
- Hummus
- Cherry tomatoes, sliced
- Feta cheese, chopped

Instructions:

- Top cucumber pieces with a spoonful of hummus.
- Add a cherry tomato half on each and sprinkle with grated feta.

Peanut Butter Banana Smoothie:

Ingredients:

- Ripe bananas
- Peanut butter
- Greek yogurt

- Almond milk
- Ice cubes

Instructions:

- Blend bananas, peanut butter, Greek yogurt, almond milk, and ice cubes until smooth.

Tomato Basil Bruschetta:

Ingredients:

- Roma tomatoes, diced
- Fresh basil, chopped
- Garlic, minced
- Olive oil
- Baguette pieces

Instructions:

- Mix tomatoes, basil, garlic, and olive oil in a bowl.
- Toast bread pieces and top with the tomato mixture.

Greek Yogurt Parfait with Berries:

Ingredients:

- Greek yogurt
- Mixed berries (strawberries, blueberries, raspberries)
- Granola

Instructions:

- Layer Greek yogurt, mixed fruit, and cereal in a glass or bowl.

Cheese and Whole Grain Crackers:

Ingredients:

- Assorted cheeses (cheddar, brie, gouda)
- Whole grain crackers
- Grapes

Instructions:

- Arrange cheese and crackers on a serving plate. Add grapes for a sweet touch.

Dark Chocolate-Dipped Almonds:

Ingredients:

- Almonds
- Dark chocolate, melted
- Sea salt

Instructions:

- Dip nuts in melted dark chocolate and sprinkle with a pinch of sea salt.
- Allow to cool until the chocolate sets.

Chapter 7: Meal Planning and Prep

Weekly Meal Planning Guide

Meal planning is a proactive approach to controlling your nutrition, ensuring that you make conscious and careful choices about what you eat throughout the week. A well-structured weekly meal plan not only promotes better eating habits but also saves time and reduces stress associated with last-minute choices.

Key Components of a Weekly Meal Planning Guide:

1. Assessment of nutritional Goals:

Begin by setting detailed nutritional goals. Whether it's weight control, increased protein intake, or incorporating more vegetables, having clear goals leads to your meal choices.

2. Create a Weekly schedule:

Utilize a schedule to plan meals for the entire week. Break down each day into breakfast, lunch, dinner, and snacks. This visual aid helps you to spread nutrients evenly and plan for variety.

3. Mix macronutrients:

Ensure a mix of macronutrients (carbohydrates, proteins, and fats) in each meal. This balance supports prolonged energy levels and general well-being.

4. Incorporate Color and range:

Aim for a colorful plate by incorporating a range of fruits and veggies. Different colors often suggest diverse nutrient profiles, giving a range of vitamins, minerals, and antioxidants.

5. Consider Portion Sizes:

Be aware of portion sizes to avoid overeating. Understanding proper serving sizes helps control calorie intake and supports weight management goals.

6. Preparation and Cooking Time:

Account for your schedule when planning meals. Quick and easy recipes may be better on busy days, while you can allocate more time for cooking on days with a lighter schedule.

7. Grocery Shopping List:

Based on your planned meals, make a thorough grocery shopping list. This reduces the chances of impulse buying and ensures you have all the necessary items on hand.

8. Batch Cooking and Leftovers:

Plan for batch cooking to make bigger amounts of meals that can be portioned and stored for later in the week. The remainder can save valuable time and reduce wasted food.

9. freedom for Treats:

Allow for freedom by adding occasional treats or favorite indulgences. This helps to keep a reasonable and sustainable approach to meal planning.

10.water Planning:

Don't forget to include water in your meal plan. Water is important for general health, and planning when to drink ensures proper hydration throughout the day.

Benefits of Weekly Meal Planning:

1. Time Savings:

Eliminate the worry of choosing what to eat each day by having a clear plan. This can save time during busy weeks.

2. Cost-Effective:

Reduce food costs by getting only what you need and minimizing food waste.

3. Nutritional responsibility:

Foster responsibility for your nutritional goals, making it easy to track and change your dietary choices.

4. Healthier Eating Habits:

Encourage healthier food choices by deliberately planning balanced and healthy meals.

Simple and Time-Saving Cooking Tips

Navigating the kitchen quickly while keeping the integrity of your meals is an art that can significantly improve your cooking experience. Here are some easy and time-saving cooking tips to improve your culinary adventures:

1. Meal Planning is Key:

Plan your meals for the week in advance. This not only helps you plan your grocery shopping but also ensures you have all the necessary ingredients at hand, lowering last-minute stress.

2. Prep Ingredients Ahead of Time:

Wash, chop, and portion out veggies, spices, and other ingredients in advance. Store them in labeled cases, making it easy to grab what you need during the cooking process.

3. Invest in Time-Saving Tools:

Utilize cooking gadgets like food processors, mandolins, or slow cookers to ease jobs such as chopping, slicing, and simmering. These tools can greatly cut prep time.

4. One-Pot Wonders:

Embrace one-pot meals that minimize the amount of plates to clean. Options like stir-fries, casseroles, and sheet pan dinners make for a delicious, well-balanced lunch without a mountain of dishes.

5. Batch Cooking for the Win:

Cook in batches and freeze parts for later. This not only saves time on future meals but also ensures you have a variety of homemade choices easily available.

6. Strategic Grocery Shopping:

Make a thorough shopping list based on your planned meals. This stops pointless trips to the store and helps you stay focused, saving both time and money.

7. Master Quick Cooking Techniques:

Learn quick cooking techniques like stir-frying, sautéing, and using high heat for faster cooking times. These methods keep the flavors of foods while reducing the time spent in the kitchen.

8. Prep Protein in Bulk:

Cook a big batch of protein (chicken, beef, tofu) at the beginning of the week. Use it as a base for different recipes, saving time on individual meal preparation.

9. Create a Well-Stocked Pantry:

Maintain a well-stocked pantry with important items like canned beans, tomatoes, pasta, and rice. This allows for quick and flexible meal ideas without frequent trips to the store.

10. Clean as You Go:

Tidy up as you cook to reduce the post-cooking mess. Wash dishes, utensils, and cutting boards as you finish using them, creating a more organized and stress-free cooking setting.

11. Optimize Oven Use:

When using the oven, prepare multiple meals simultaneously to make the most of your cooking time. Ensure that things with similar cooking temperatures are put together.

Grocery Shopping Tips for Seniors

In the hustle and bustle of daily life, making nutritious meals efficiently is a common struggle. Adopting easy and time-saving cooking tips can make the kitchen a more efficient and fun place. Here are some useful ideas to streamline your cooking process:

1. Meal Planning is Key:
    - Plan your weekly meals to reduce last-minute choices and food store trips.
    - Designate specific days for batch cooking or making flexible ingredients that can be used in multiple recipes.
2. Prep Ingredients in Batches:
    - Chop veggies, marinate proteins, and measure out spices in bigger amounts.
    - Store prepped items in portioned containers for easy access during the week.
3. Invest in Time-Saving Appliances:
    - Utilize kitchen gadgets like food processors, slow cookers, or Instant Pots to expedite cooking.
    - These appliances can handle certain chores quickly, allowing you to focus on other aspects of the meal.

4. One-Pan Wonders:
   - Opt for one-pan or one-pot recipes to reduce cleanup time.
   - Roasting vegetables alongside proteins or making a sheet pan meal can ease the cooking process.
5. Master One-Pot Meals:
   - Explore recipes that can be made in a single pot or pan.
   - Dishes like casseroles, stir-fries, or soups often take less hands-on time and result in fewer dishes to wash.
6. Pre-Cut and Frozen Ingredients:
   - Purchase pre-cut veggies or frozen options to save time on chopping.
   - Frozen fruits and vegetables can be just as nutritious and are useful for quick additions to recipes.
7. Organize Your cooking:
   - Arrange your cooking tools and utensils carefully for easy access.
   - Keep frequently used items within reach to reduce search time during cooking.
8. Cook Once, Eat Twice:
   - Prepare bigger numbers of meals and freeze leftovers for future quick and easy meals.
   - This method can save time and ensure you always have a homemade choice on hand.
9. Multi-Task Efficiently:

- Identify jobs that can be done jointly. For example, chop veggies while water is boiling or use oven time to make side dishes.
- Be aware of overlapping jobs to improve your time in the kitchen.

10. Embrace Shortcut Ingredients:
- Use comfort items like pre-cooked grains, canned beans, or store-bought sauces to cut down on cooking time.
- Check for high-quality, healthy options to keep the nutritional worth of your meals.

Chapter 8: Success Stories and Testimonials

Real-life Experiences of Seniors Who Benefited from the Cookbook

Within the pages of the "Belly Fat Busters for Seniors Cookbook," real-life stories unfold, creating a patchwork of motivation and change. These tales shine a light on the tangible effect that adopting healthier eating habits can have on the lives of seniors.

1. Meet Helen, 68:

Helen, after years of battling with extra weight and low energy, found the recipe and decided to give it a try. By adding delicious recipes and nutritional insights into her daily routine, she not only shed unwanted belly fat but also experienced a newfound vigor. Helen's story connects with those wanting a fresh start in their golden years.

2. John's Journey, 73:

John, a testament to the cookbook's practicality, found joy in creating the recipes suited for seniors. His favorites included the Turkey and Vegetable Stir-Fry and the Nut and Seed Trail Mix. John's success not only shows in his physical well-being but also in the delight he now finds in cooking and enjoying nutritious meals.

3. Mary's Thoughtful Eating, 70:

For Mary, the recipe became a guide to thoughtful eating. Struggling with portion control and mindless eating, she found a treasure trove of tips and tricks within its pages. Through the suggested meal planning and portion control techniques, Mary not only achieved her weight management goals but also fostered a better relationship with food.

4. Richard's Heart-Healthy Choices, 75:

Richard, aware of his heart health, found comfort in the cookbook's focus on heart-healthy ingredients. By adding lean proteins, smart carbs, and healthy fats to his meals, Richard not only experienced a reduction in belly fat but also noticed positive changes in his cholesterol levels. His story echoes the cookbook's approach to promoting overall well-being.

5. Eleanor's Culinary Journey, 72:

Eleanor, an active senior with a love for trying new recipes, found the guide to be a fascinating culinary journey. The varied range of recipes, from Greek Yogurt Parfait to Vegetarian Chili with Beans and Greens, offered Eleanor a variety of choices to keep her meals interesting and filling.

Chapter 9: Conclusion

As we conclude the "Belly Fat Busters for Seniors Cookbook," it's an ideal moment to reflect on the transforming journey started within these pages. This cookbook, created with the well-being of adults in mind, goes beyond being a mere collection of recipes. It serves as a complete guide, enabling you to take charge of your health, reshape your physique, and enjoy the golden years with energy and joy.

Recap of Key Concepts:

In the chapters preceding this conclusion, we explored the importance of healthy eating for seniors, dove into nutritional basics, found belly fat-busting ingredients, and delighted in delicious and healthy recipes. We found the importance of smart carbohydrate choices, reviewed tips for healthy living, and even went into the realms of meal planning and preparation.

Encouragement for a Healthy Lifestyle: The recipes and directions shared are not merely a short fix but a sustainable approach to better living. Whether you found comfort in the ease of a fiber-packed smoothie or the heartiness of a vegetarian chili, each recipe is a stepping stone toward a more vibrant you. The encouragement to make smart food choices, value regular exercise and handle stress echoes throughout these pages.

Closing Thoughts:

As you bid farewell to this cookbook, know that your road toward health and well-being is continuing. Embrace the small wins, enjoy your progress, and savor the joys that follow a healthy lifestyle. The power to change your health and shape lies within your choices, and this cookbook has provided you with the tools to make those choices wisely.

May the recipes, insights, and support found in the "Belly Fat Busters for Seniors Cookbook" continue to serve as a source of inspiration as you travel the path to a better, more satisfying life. Here's to welcoming your golden years with renewed energy, nourishment, and a deep sense of well-being. Cheers to your health and happiness!

www.ingramcontent.com/pod-product-compliance
Lightning Source LLC
Chambersburg PA
CBHW061016260726
48661CB00005B/2212